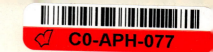

HERBS FOR
FEMININE AILMENTS

145

By the same author
HERBS FOR CLEARING THE SKIN
HERBS TO SOOTHE YOUR NERVES

HERBS FOR
FEMININE AILMENTS

by
SARAH BECKETT

Drawings by Jill Fry

THORSONS PUBLISHERS LIMITED
Denington Estate, Wellingborough
Northamptonshire

First published August 1973

ISBN 0 7225 0213 3

Typesetting by
Specialised Offset Services Limited, Liverpool
Made and printed in Great Britain by
Weatherby Woolnough Ltd., Sanders Road,
Wellingborough, Northants

CONTENTS

SOME FACTS ABOUT WOMEN'S DISEASES

Owing to present-day conditions and modes of life, many women suffer symptoms in the pelvic region which they accept as normal. It should, however, be stressed from the beginning that the sexual and reproductive organs play a decisive and important role in the life of every woman; their functions are natural and rhythmical and should cause no pain or discomfort.

Let us first try to understand what menstruation is all about. A girl's digestion and assimilation are arranged in order that for some thirty-five years, that is from puberty to the menopause, sufficient blood is made for her own use and activities plus some which should, or might, be needed for producing and feeding a baby. Menstruation is primarily to maintain a balance by discharging blood that is not required in the unmarried girl, or later, if pregnancy does not take place. But that is not all. The menses act as a purifier of the blood and each month many poisons are cast out with the flow. This is one of the reasons why it is so important that a woman should have a regular and normal menstruation.

In adolescence, menses — or periods — can begin at the early age of eleven years but more often a girl is twelve or thirteen before the breasts begin to fill out and the first flow commences.

At the beginning of menstruation, periods are often irregular for a month or two but gradually, without anything being done, the cycle becomes rhythmical and all is well.

Occasionally menses do not commence in a teenager and steps have to be taken to remedy what is known as amenorrhoea. On the other hand, sometimes regular periods stop for one reason or another; pregnancy is excluded at this point. This may be caused by an operation, a serious illness, a bad chill or exposure to cold. or the cause could be due to disease of the sexual organs. If the latter is the case treatment is necessary and the sooner the better. This cessation could be due to a sudden shock, worry, anxiety or an emotional upset and whilst it is possible that the regular cycle may return, help may be needed, and the cause taken into consideration.

Irregularity of the menses is another symptom common to many women. Instead of a usual cycle of 28 days (it can vary a little according to individual idiosyncrasy), the time in between the flow can alter from month to month, sometimes quite considerably. Apart from the inconvenience, this is a symptom that all is not well and steps should be taken to cure it.

Dysmenorrhoea or painful menstruation is often complained of and is usually worst during the first day or two of the period, but some women experience bad pains for two or three days before it commences. They may be accompanied by sickness or a feeling of nausea, sometimes headaches develop, and if very bad the sufferer has to retire to bed for a few hours. For some, this malaise is the forerunner of each monthly period.

The flow can vary considerably. It can be scanty or profuse; very heavy for one or two days and then trickle on for several more; it may be clotted and it is sometimes thin and pale in colour.

Some women are affected emotionally each month, and may become irritable, weepy, short-tempered or indifferent. Generally these states do not last very long and often disappear as soon as the flow begins.

But again, it should be emphasized that the monthly cycle is a natural rhythm of the body and any abnormalities should be put right to ensure the health of every woman.

The menopause, known as 'change of life' or 'climacteric' usually takes place between the age of forty-five to fifty years, when the menses stop. This happens in a gradual way for most women, although a sudden ending can occur. Many women are affected emotionally and some go through a very difficult time, feeling nervy and on edge, indifferent to their family and friends and even fearful of going out on their own; others seek company all the time. They can be weepy and fearful and quite different from their normal personalities.

One of the most common and inconvenient post-menopausal troubles is hot-flushes from which many women suffer, and some for a long period.

There is a school of thought (with which the author agrees), that when periods cease, the poisons from the body can no longer be thrown out at monthly intervals, and therefore there has to be a complete readjustment to cope with this situation. Once again it must be stated that the menopause is another natural function and there are many women who feel no ill effects at all, but if symptoms do appear, then treatment should be given to help the body to readjust and so ward off any chronic diseases developing in later years.

Leucorrhoea or 'whites' is a discharge from the vagina which is really a catarrh. It can be very profuse, of a creamy yellow or even brownish colour, thickish or almost like coloured water. It occurs most frequently up to the age of thirty-five years although it can go on and sometimes continues after the menopause. Leucorrhoea should never be suppressed or neglected as it is an outlet for poisons; and it may be a sign that all is not well with the pelvic organs themselves, particularly if it continues after the menopause.

Some women suffer from prolapse or displacement of the uterus or womb. The virgin womb, if healthy, is rather like a large inverted pear, which balloons about within the pelvic structure out of harm's way. When the organ becomes sick, in other words heavy, enlarged or displaced, it drops down or tips over on its side and becomes uncomfortable. The use of pessaries or the intervention of surgery is not wholly satisfactory; how can it be when the organ itself needs attention to help it to return to its normal weight and buoyancy? This can be achieved in many cases with the help of herbal remedies which are discussed later.

And finally, much can be done to help the expectant mother through the nine months of pregnancy, and to ensure that the actual birth is as easy as possible. In very many cases raspberry leaf tea has made this event much more normal and less painful than most mothers-to-be think possible, for let us not lose sight of the fact that this too is a natural event and not to be dreaded, as is sometimes the case.

If at any time organic change is suspected, then a qualified medical herbalist or local doctor should be consulted at once.

Many symptoms common to women are caused by toxic conditions, unhealthy living, a refined diet and lack of exercise. This is discussed, and help given in the section on supplementary advice.

2
SOME THOUGHTS ABOUT HERBAL MEDICINES

There is no doubt that herbal remedies offer a means whereby many of the aches and pains suffered by women can be dealt with satisfactorily in the home. A great deal can be done to eradicate that which is wrong and so promote better health and well-being.

Quotations from old herbals help us to understand that in days gone by the herbalists did amazing work with their plants, and it is hoped that more and more people will turn once again to healing by nature's safe methods.

A question may come to mind when reading that one herb will not only help suppressed menses but also reduce a profuse flow! The answer is really quite a simple one. Herbs contain many substances such as minerals, vitamins and oils, etc., all in their natural form, and when taken into the body they correct imbalances, create order out of chaos, and when harmony is restored, health returns and symptoms vanish. And we must never forget that when herbs are used there are no side effects.

The relaxing herbs help the cramping pains which often accompany the monthly period, and others cleanse the blood stream and clear up the discharges which occur in between the menstrual flow or after the menopause, (leucorrhoea). As was explained in the previous section, this is a catarrhal state and many herbs have done good work in curing this condition.

At the time of the menopause many women have been more than grateful for the way in which herbs have helped to smooth the path through a difficult time. Some women get very frustrated and upset mentally, in fact they can be quite unlike themselves, but herbs can help to readjust and restore harmony and all is well once more.

Some cases of prolapse of the uterus respond to herbal treatment, although this may take time, but if the organ and muscle structures in the pelvic girdle can regain their tone, then the womb will become lighter and be supported in its natural position. This is not always possible, particularly in the case of older women, but a course of herbal medicines is well worth trying.

During the nine months of pregnancy, herbs can play their part, particularly raspberry leaf tea, full details of which are given later in this book. It is of great importance in helping the actual birth by relaxing the muscles and so making delivery as easy as possible.

It must be reiterated that herbs do more than remove symptoms; they restore balance and harmony in the patient and thus raise vitality and the level of health.

After reading some of the books in 'Everybody's Home Herbal' series it is hoped that many people will make, and take, infusions or teas from herbs according to their symptoms, and adopt a new way of life as described in the section headed Supplementary Advice. In so doing there is no doubt that some benefits will be derived and a greater sense of well-being experienced.

ANGELICA
(Angelica archangelica)

Also known as Garden angelica and Master-wort.

Description: It is common in gardens in England and it also grows wild. The plant grows to about 6 feet tall on large hollow stems, the bottom leaves are large, broad and pointed with serrated edges, on short stalks. The upper leaves are similar but smaller. There are large heads made up of tiny greenish-white flowers. The root is from 2 to 4 inches long and 1 to 2 inches thick; when cut the fresh root yields a thick yellow juice. The smell is fragrant, the taste aromatic.

Part used: Root, seeds and herb, but mostly an infusion from the herb.

The fruit of Angelica is used for flavouring the liqueur Chartreuse and the stems are candied and used in cake making and to decorate trifles, etc.

It is said that Archangelica was revealed in a dream by an angel to cure the plague; others insist that it blooms on the day of Michael the Archangel and is a preservative against evil spirits and witchcraft.

Salmon says, 'It provokes urine and the courses and expels both birth and afterbirth'.

It is excellent for both suppressed and delayed menstruation, it also expels afterbirth.

Directions for use: 1 pint of boiling water should be poured on to 1 oz. of the powdered root, and a wineglassful taken hot, three times daily. The same directions should be used but substituting 1 oz. of the dried herb for the powdered root; it should be taken in the same way.

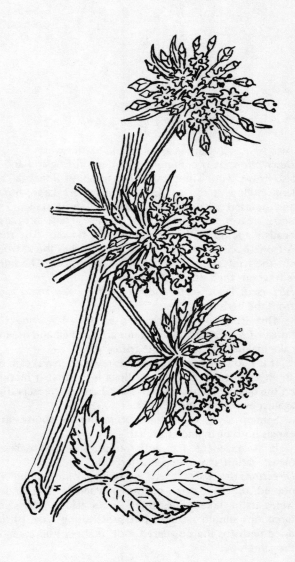

ARRACH
(Chenopodium olidum)

Also known as Stinking Arrach, Stinking Goosefoot, Dog's Arrach, Goat's Arrach, Stinking Motherwort.

Description: This herb is found in waste places and particularly on dunghills. It grows near the ground with fleshy oval leaves, notched near the base; the underside is covered in greasy meal, which gives off a very odious smell like that of stale fish which remains on the hands after washing. The greenish yellow flowers grow in clusters at the base of the leaves.

Part used: The herb.

The name Chenopodium is derived from the Greek word *chen*, a goose, and *pous*, a foot, because the leaves bear a resemblance to the webbed feet of 'that waddling bird' which, says Fernie, 'raw recruits are wont to bless for their irksome drill of the goose step'.

Culpeper has been quoted often in this series but rather more of what he says about this herb is given as it is so quaint and in some places amusing. 'Stinking arrach is used as a remedy to help women pained, and almost strangled with the mother by smelling to it; but inwardly taken there is no better remedy under the moon for that disease. I would be large in commendation of this herb, were I but eloquent. It is an herb under the dominion of Venus and under the sign of Scorpio; it is common almost upon every dunghill. The works of God are given freely to man, his medicines are common and cheap and easy to be found ('Tis the medicines of the College of Physicians that are so dear and scarce to find.) I commend it for a universal medicine of the womb, and such a medicine as will easily, safely and speedily cure any disease thereof; as fits of the mother, dislocation, or falling out thereof; it cools the womb being overheated. And let me tell you this, and I will tell you the truth — heat of the womb is one of the greatest causes of hard labour in child-birth. It makes barren women fruitful: it cleanseth the womb if it be foul, and strengthens it exceedingly; it provokes the terms if they be stopped and stops them if they flow immoderately; you can desire no good to your womb but this herb will affect it; therefore if you love children, if you love health, if you love ease, keep a syrup always by you made of the juice of this herb, and sugar, or honey, if it be to cleanse the womb and let such as be rich keep it for their poor neighbours, and bestow it as freely as I bestow my studies upon them, or else let them look to answer it another day, when the Lord shall come to make the inquisition of blood.'

This is an excellent herb to control the menses, whether they be too profuse or suppressed. It is also very good in the hysteria of women which often coincides with this irregularity.

Directions for use: An infusion is made by pouring 1 pint of boiling water on to 1 oz. of the dried herb, when cold this should be strained and a wineglassful taken three or four times daily.

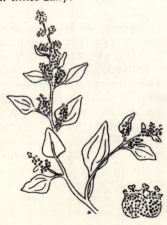

BALM
(Melissa officinalis)

Also known as Sweet Balm, Lemon Balm, Honey Plant, Cure-All.

Description: This is a common plant which often grows in cottage gardens, but was originally the wild 'bastard balm' growing in woods especially in Southern England. The leaves grow opposite, are dark green, serrated and wrinkled. Small white flowers grow very near the stem. It tastes and smells like lemons.

Part used: The whole herb.

In olden days this herb was known as Bawme. In his herbal of 1710 Salmon says, 'It causes speedy and easie delivery to women in travel . . . It may be profitably given to women in child-bed, to bring away the after-birth, or cause a perfect cleansing'.

Culpeper says ' . . . and commendeth the decoction for women to bathe or sit in to procure their courses . . . A tansy or caudle made with eggs and juice thereof, while it is young, putting to some sugar and rose-water, is good for a woman in childbed when the after-birth is not thoroughly voided, and for their faintings upon, or in their sore travail'.

And in France, we are told, women used to bruise the young shoots of balm and make them into cakes with eggs, sugar and rose-water, which they gave to mothers in child bed or as a strengthener.

Balm is excellent for delayed menstruation, especially if caused by a chill. It also helps considerably the pains before and during periods, if taken hot as a tea, and is good for suppressed menses.

Directions for use: An infusion is made by pouring a pint of boiling water on to 1 oz. of the fresh or dried herb. When cold this should be strained and a wine-glassful taken three times daily.

A tea may be made by adding a pint of boiling water to two teaspoonsful of the balm. This should infuse for about five minutes and then be taken as a tea. It may be sweetened with a little honey if desired.

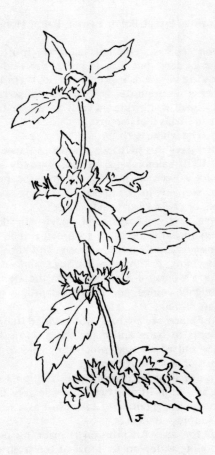

BASIL
(Ocimum basilicum)

Also known as Sweet Basil, Garden Basil.

Description: This plant is an annual but is planted every year in many English gardens. It grows about 8 inches high, and usually has one upright branched stem. The leaves grow opposite on short stalks, broad, oval and pointed. The flowers are small, white with purple, in long, loose spikes. It has an aromatic taste.

Part used: The herb.

An old writer says this herb is so called because 'the smell thereof is fit for a king's house'. When bruised, the leaves of sweet basil give off a delightful odour.

Dr Fernie tells us, 'Its seed were sown by the Romans with maledictions and curses under the belief that the more it was abused the better it would prosper. When desiring a good crop they trod it down with their feet and prayed the gods it might not vegetate'.

And Culpeper says, 'This is the herb which all authors are together by the ears about, and rail at one another, like lawyers! and something is the matter; basil and rue, will never grow together nor near each other'.

Basil will relieve pains caused by delayed menses, and a tea taken hot, will help when they are suppressed.

Directions for use: A pint of boiling water should be poured on to two teaspoonsful of the dried herb and after infusing for five minutes, it should be taken as tea.

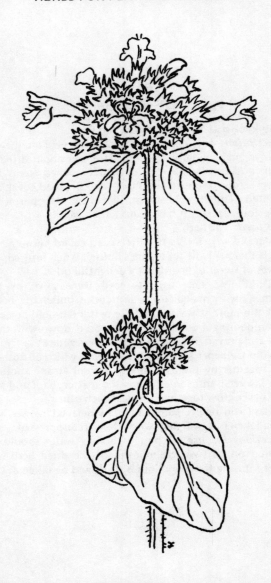

BLACK COHOSH
(Cimicifuga racemosa)

Also known as Black snakeroot, Bugbane, Rattleroot, Rattleweed, Squawroot.

Description: Black cohosh grows in herbaceous borders so long as it has plenty of sunshine, but its home is America, Canada and Kashmir. It has snake-like cream flowers and the root is thick, hard and knotty with short lateral branches.

Part used: The root.

It is very valuable for its action on the pelvic structures and particularly uterine disturbances. It relieves neuralgia and rheumatic pains in this area very promptly. It is helpful in prolapse of the uterus and also leucorrhoea accompanied by a sense of weight in the uterus.

In suppressed menses, with pain in back, pelvis and thighs, particularly when caused by exposure to damp or cold, a hot infusion is excellent.

A case comes to mind of a young woman of twenty-three who was very worried as her periods had stopped. At first she said she could not account for this but when questioned closely she remembered being caught in a very heavy rainstorm and being thoroughly soaked. Instead of going home and getting into a warm bath, she called to see a relative and as it was late when she arrived home she went to bed. Suppression of her menses was the outcome. She had black cohosh for just over two weeks when her period returned and sub-sequently was quite regular.

This herb is very good for irregular, or scanty menses with muscular soreness, dragging pains with soreness, and when pains come immediately before the flow of blood.

Directions for use: 10-15 drops of the fluid extract should be taken in water three times daily for two or three weeks.

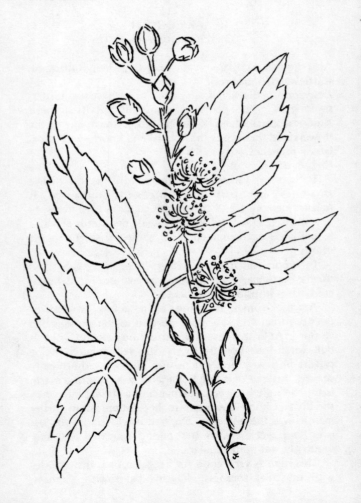

BLACK HOREHOUND
(Ballota nigra)

Also known as Madwort.

Description: It is a common herb found growing in hedgerows and on waste land. The leaves are ovate, two growing at a joint opposite each other on leaf stalks, dented at the edges, dark green on top, paler underneath, with netted veins and slightly hairy. The stem grows from 1 to 4 feet. The flowers grow in whorls, the calyx being funnel-shaped, with short, spreading teeth and dilated at the mouth. The corolla is dark purple, the upper lip cleft and is covered with small white hairs. It has a disagreeable odour.

Part used: The leaves.

Of this herb Anne Pratt says, 'It is not often seen in woods and hedges far away from houses; but there are few English villages or towns, except in Scotland and Ireland, in or near which we might not find it. It is one of those plants which follow man, and besides being pretty general all over Europe, it is to be found in Australia wherever the English colonist has come, and the Horehound raises its tall stem by many of the sheep stations of that country'.

The Swedes think it a remedy for almost every disease to which cattle are liable.

In suppressed and also in excessive menstruation it is extremely helpful. It may seem contradictory to say that this herb may be prescribed in what are generally considered to be opposite conditions of the system; but when it is understood that in either case the disturbance of the physiological condition is simply due to a loss of equilibrium and that the black horehound exerts such an influence that will restore the necessary balance, it will

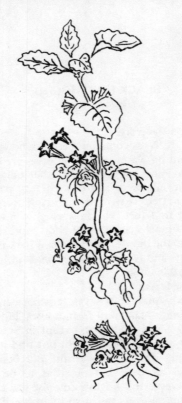

be realized that it is equally applicable in either case.

Culpeper says, 'It is a promoter of the menses'.

In the pains of labour, combined with motherwort, it will be found an excellent remedy.

Directions for use: A pint of boiling water should be poured on to 1 oz. of the leaves, strained when cold, and a wineglassful taken three times daily. When used with motherwort, a pint of boiling water should be poured on to ½ oz. leaves of black horehound plus ½ oz. motherwort. Half a teacupful of the hot infusion should be taken frequently for labour pains.

CATMINT
(Nepita cataria)

Also known as Catnep or Nep.

Description: This herb grows in hedgerows and on waste ground and has become a common garden plant. It is 2 to 3 feet in height; the stems are square and at every junction there are two broad leaves, covered with down, nicked at the edges and aromatic. The flowers are purple-white and grow in tufts at the top of the branches and lower down the stems. The stems and leaves are so covered with down, they look white.

Part used: The herb.

Several kinds of the Mints have been used medicinally from the earliest times, such as balm, basil, ground ivy, horehound, marjoram, pennyroyal, peppermint, rosemary, sage, savory, spearmint and thyme; and to a lesser degree catmint and horsemint.

Dr Fernie tells us, 'They have acquired their common name "Mentha" from Minthes (according to Ovid) who was changed into a plant of this sort by Proserpina, the wife of Pluto, in a fit of jealousy'.

Culpeper says, 'It is a herb of Venus and is generally used to procure women's courses, taken outwardly or inwardly, either alone or with other convenient herbs in a decoction to bathe them or sit over the hot fumes; and by frequent use it takes away barrenness, the wind and pains of the mother'.

This herb is a splendid antispasmodic and nervine and is excellent in the treatment of dysmenorrhoea (difficult menstruation).

It is most helpful when there is nervous agitation preceding menses in weak and very excitable women when the flow is tardy and sluggish.

Directions for use: A tea is made by pouring a pint of boiling water on to 2 teaspoonsful of the dried herb and allowing it to infuse for five minutes. This should be taken hot and may be sweetened with a little honey if desired. Make in a teapot, as it is better not exposed to the air.

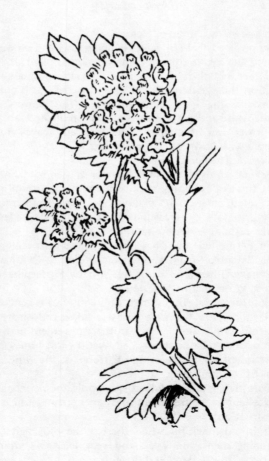

CRAMP BARK
(Viburnum opulus)

Also known as Guelder Rose, High Cranberry, Dogberry, Snowball tree.

Description: This grows to a large shrub and can be about 10 feet tall in Britain, with lovely sweet-smelling white flowers which, from a distance, look very like snowballs. The bark is very thin, greyish-brown.

Part used: The bark.

This shrub was first grown in Holland, hence its name Guelder Rose.

As its name suggests cramp bark is a relaxant, and so cures cramps. Therefore it is very helpful in the cramping pains of pregnancy which often occur in the legs and calves.

It is excellent in difficult and painful menstruation when there are bearing down and neuralgic pains of the uterus (possibly caused by a chill), with cold extremities. Cramp bark relaxes the ovaries and again helps in painful menses.

In any spasmodic, cramping pains at the time of the menses, this herb should be remembered.

Directions for use: 1 pint of water should be poured on to ½ oz. of the powdered root and a wineglassful taken three times daily, or when required.

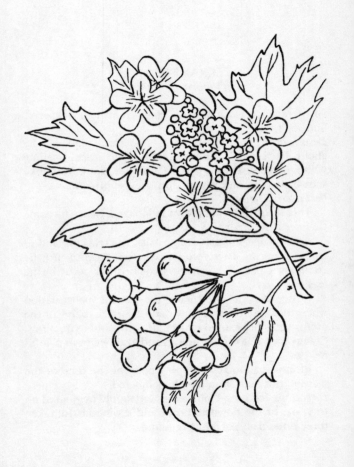

FENNEL
(Foeniculum officinalis)

Also known as Hinojo.

Description: This plant grows wild on waste ground and near the sea on cliff tops. It is 4 to 5 feet tall, having feathery leaves with yellow flowers borne in large terminals, followed by fruits, long and oval, blunt at the ends with eight longitudinal ridges.

Part used: The fruit.

An old herbalist wrote, 'Every garden affordeth this so plentifully that it needs no description', and he goes on, 'one good old fashion is not yet left off, viz. to boil fennel with fish', and I suspect that it is with fish we all connect the herb fennel!

Parkinson wrote of it in 1629, 'Fennel is useful to strowe upon fish, as also to boyle and put among fish of divers sorts', and he adds, 'Cocumbers and other fruits are picked with it and the seedes are much used to be put in Pippin Pies, and divers other such baked fruits as also into bread to give it a better relish'.

The accounts of Edward 1, for the year 1281 show that eight-and-a-half pounds of seed were bought for one month's supply for the Royal household!

The Greeks of olden times held it in high esteem for promoting the milk in nursing mothers.

Culpeper says, 'The leaves or seed boiled in barley water and drunk are good for nurses to increase their milk and make it more wholesome for the child'.

Fernie says that an hot infusion made by pouring half a pint of boiling water on a teaspoonful of the bruised seeds will prove an active remedy in promoting monthly regularity, if taken at the periodical times, in doses of a wineglassful three times daily.

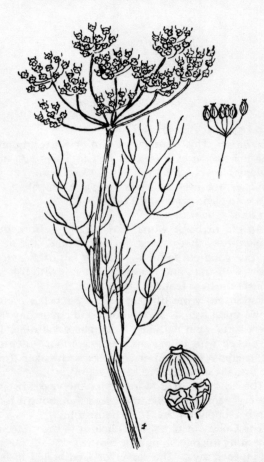

And Gerard says, 'The green leaves of the fennel eaten, or the seed made into a ptisan and drunk, do fill women's breasts with milk'.

This culinary herb will increase the menstrual flow.

Directions for use: Make and drink it as a tea by infusing two teaspoonsful of the powdered seeds with a pint of boiling water, then leave to steep for five minutes.

FEVERFEW
(Chrysanthemum parthenium)

Also known as Pyrethrum parthenium, Featherfew, Featherfoil, Bachelor's buttons, Maydeweed.

Description: This plant grows from 1 to 2 feet high in every hedgerow and the stalked leaves are feathery and of a delicate green. They are downy, about 4½ inches long and 2 inches broad. The flower stalks are branched, and the disk-flowers are yellow with short white rays around.

Part used: The herb.

The whole plant emits an aromatic pungent scent when handled and people who are afraid of bees should carry a sprig as these insects dislike feverfew.

The name is a corruption of 'Febrifuga' from its old uses in fevers. It is known as featherfew because of the feathery appearance of the leaves, which retain their lovely bright colour during the winter months.

Culpeper says, 'Venus commands this herb and has commended it to succour her sisters (women) to be a general strengthener of their wombs, and to remedy such affirmities as a careless midwife has there caused; if they will be pleased to make use of her herb boiled in white wine and drunk in decoction, it cleanses the womb, expels the afterbirth and does a woman all the good she can desire of an herb'.

This is a splendid herb for promoting the menses, especially if the patient is hysterical; or if she is chilly and suffers from headaches.

Directions for use: An infusion is made by pouring 1 pint of boiling water on to 1 oz. of the dried herb; this can be taken frequently in half-teacupful doses.

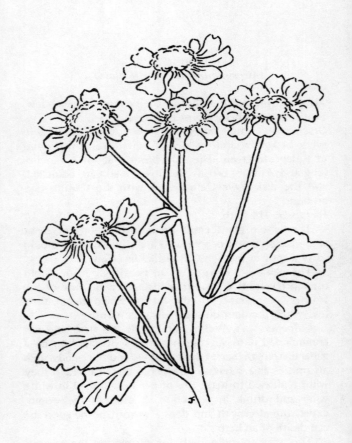

LADY'S SLIPPER
(Cypripedum pubescens)

Also known as Lady's shoe, Nerve-root, Noah's Ark, Yellow Lady's Slipper.

Description: This is one of the rarest and most beautiful of the British wild flowers; it is now almost extinct except in Yorkshire and Durham. It has a creeping root from which a downy stalk rises to about 12 inches. The leaves are broad, pale green and heavily ribbed and there are three or four on each stem. At the top of the stem there is one flower with reddish, sometimes twisted sepals, and a large yellow lip which attracts the bees. The flowers are large and showy and when newly open they have a very soft perfume.

Part used: The root.

This is an excellent herb for women having a bad time during the menopause. The symptoms to look for are certain fears, particularly of disaster; a patient who worries about everything, and the hypochondriac who thinks of nothing much else but her own troubles, whether they are real or imagined.

It is a 'relaxant' and therefore will help the cramping pains before and during menses.

Directions for use: An infusion should be made by pouring 1 pint of boiling water on to 1 oz. of the powdered root and strained when cold. A wineglassful should be taken three times daily.

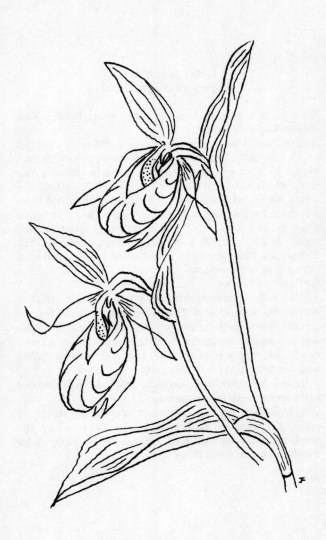

MOTHERWORT
(*Leonurus cardiaca*)

Also known as Lion's ear, Lion's tail.

Description: This herb grows wild in Britain and commonly in gardens. The stem is square growing to 3 feet, spreading into many branches, the lower leaves are five lobed and the upper three lobed, two leaves grow at every joint. The flowers grow in dense whorls in the axils of the upper leaves, white or pink, purple spotted. It has an aromatic odour when bruised.

Part used: The herb.

Its name of 'Cardiaca' was given because the plant was formerly supposed to cure, not only heart-burn, but the mental malady figuratively called heart-ache!

Culpeper says ' . . . it makes mothers joyful and settles the womb, therefore it is called Motherwort. It provokes urine and women's courses'.

And Salmon says, 'It is effectual against all sorts of bleeding both inward and outward. It stops the overflowing of the Terms in Women . . . and is a peculiar thing to stop the Whites in women, being esteemed more powerful for this purpose than most other things . . . The essence being taken for twenty or thirty days together by such Women as are Barren, or have a Slipperiness of the Womb, it is said to cause them to Conceive, and to retain the birth after Conception'.

This is an excellent herb for all female troubles and it acts as a general tonic to debilitated generative organs with discomfort and bearing down pains, and allays nervous irritability. It would benefit sufferers from prolapse troubles.

It is used with very good results in suppressed menses: and it increases the flow.

It tones up the uterine membranes.

Directions for use: An infusion is made by pouring 1 pint of boiling water on to 1 oz. of the herb and when cold this should be strained and a wineglassful taken three times daily. An hot fomentation wrung out of a strong tea (half a pint of boiling water poured on 1 oz. of the herb), will relieve cramps and pain in painful menstruation.

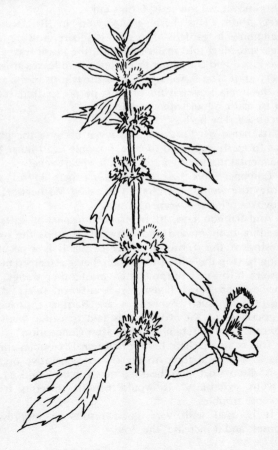

MUGWORT
(Artemisia vulgaris)

Also known as Felon Herb.

Description: This herb is found growing by the roadside on rubbish heaps and by the side of rivers, etc. It is a common plant and grows all over Britain, on a stem 3 to 6 feet high, erect, the dark green leaves deeply incised, with sharply serrated teeth, silvery white underneath from the downy hairs. The leaves grow alternately. The flowers grow up the main stem and on branches rather like yellow-brown buttons.

Parts used: The leaves and flowers.

Fernie tells us that the name 'mugwort' has been attributed to 'moughte' a moth or maggot, this title being given to the plant because Dioscorides commended it for keeping off moths. But it may be because this herb was in demand for helping to preserve ale.

The plant was formerly known as Cingulum Sancti Johannis as a crown made from its sprays was worn on St John's eve, to gain security from evil possession.

Pliny said, 'The traveller or wayfaring man that hath the herb tied about him feeleth no weariness at all; and he can never be hurt by poisonous medicine, by any wild beast, neither by the sun itself'.

In former days it was placed in baths and thought to have great effect in relieving fatigue; and the pilgrim used to place it in his shoes, in full faith in its efficacy to strengthen him.

Parkinson says, 'Mugwort is of wonderful help to women in risings of the mother or hysteria'.

Salmon says, 'It provokes the Terms powerfully and facilitates the Birth of Women in labour bringing away After Birth and causing a due cleansing'.

This is an excellent female medicine and may be relied upon in obstructed menstruation, particularly if from cold.

It is also very good for young girls when their periods are not regular, or when there is any suppression of menses it is a very safe remedy. It is excellent too when there are contractions of the uterus and spasms of pain during menses.

Directions for use: An infusion is made by pouring 1 pint of boiling water on to 1 oz. of the dried leaves and flowers and steeped for 20 minutes. For suppressed menses a wineglassful should be taken three times a day for a week before the period is due. Otherwise a wineglassful should be taken twice daily plus half a teacupful at bedtime, taken hot.

This may also be taken as a tea. Add 1 pint of boiling water to 2 teaspoonsful of the herb, let it stand for four minutes before pouring. A little honey may be used to sweeten.

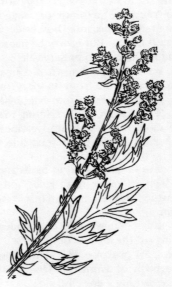

PEPPERMINT
(Mentha peperita)

Also called Brandy mint, Balm mint, Curled mint.

Description: Peppermint is found in many European countries and is often cultivated in our country gardens. It grows on a purplish stem from 2 to 3 feet high, with stalked leaves 2-3 inches long and 1-1½ inches broad with a serrated edge; slightly hairy. The flowers are numerous, purplish in colour, and grow in loose spikes on top of the branches. Both leaves and flowers have a pleasant scent, and a hot, biting taste like pepper.

Part used: The herb, distilled oil.

Pliny tells us that the Greeks and Romans crowned themselves with Peppermint at their feasts, and adorned their al fresco tables with its sprays. The chefs introduced this herb into all their sauces, and scented their wines with its essence. The Roman housewives made a paste of the Peppermint with honey, which they esteemed highly, partaking of it to sweeten their breath, and to conceal their passion for wine at a time when the law punished with death, every woman convicted of quaffing the seductive ruby liquor.

Fernie says, 'Preparations of peppermint when swallowed, diffuse warmth in the stomach and mouth, acting as a stimulating carminative (a medicine which removes wind and flatus from stomach and intestines) with some amount of anodyne power to allay the pain of colic, flatulence, spasm, or indigestion. This is through the powerful volatile oil of which the herb yields one per cent'.

Peppermint is very beneficial for acute internal pains from suppressed menses and also for headaches from the same cause.

It is a most useful medicine when there has been a cessation of menses for sometime with pallor of the cheeks; especially when the patient takes cold easily; there may be anaemia and langour, and most probably dark circles under the eyes with pains in the back.

Directions for use: The best way is to make peppermint tea by adding 1 pint of boiling water to 2 teaspoonsful of the dried herb, which is put into a teapot. Allow to infuse for about five minutes and then drink as tea as often as required, or three times daily. It may be slightly sweetened if desired, with honey or brown sugar.

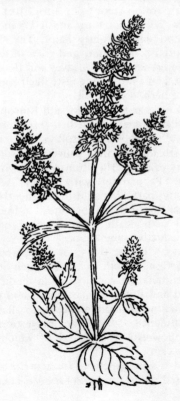

PULSATILLA
(Anemone pulsatilla)

Also known as Pasque flower, Passe flower, Easter flower, Wind flower, Blue money, Blue anemone, Flaw flower.

Description: It grows on chalky pasture land and has a stout woody root stock that runs deep into the earth to allow it to get moisture in the calcareous soil. It throws up stalks of 6-8 inches and has a quantity of leaves very like those of a carrot. When young they have many silky hairs as do the flowers, stalks and buds. As a bud opens, a large and very handsome flower comes forth, of dark purple and bright yellow. It has a ring of six petal-like sepals of dark purple, richly coloured on the inside but shining with a silky coat on the back. The stamens are brilliant yellow.

Part used: The herb.

The name Pulsatilla is from the Latin *Puls*, a pottage made from pulse and used at sacrificial feasts. Anemone signifies 'windflower' and it is said that this plant only opens its flowers when the wind is blowing. It is also called the Passover flower because it has been connected with Eastertide since olden days, and is in bloom at that time.

Salmon says, ' . . . but is chiefly given inwardly to provoke the terms, bring away the birth, after-birth or dead child'.

This herb is used much more for women than for men, and it suits best those who have a gentle disposition and who weep easily although other temperaments have also derived benefit from it.

It is excellent for amenorrhoea, tardy or insufficient menses with a sense of fulness in the pelvic area and

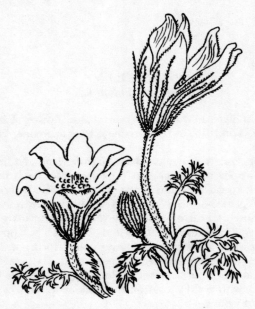

weakness of back and loins; and there is very often chilliness and depression.

It helps painful and difficult menstruation when the patient is chilly and feels very gloomy.

Pulsatilla helps to clear up leucorrhoea which is profuse, thick, milky, yellow, or bland, with often a pain in the loins.

It should be thought of for nervous exhaustion in women due to any menstrual troubles.

Pulsatilla has helped to restore the uterus to normality after a prolapsed condition in some cases, especially in women with dispositions as described above. It helps women who are going through the menopause when there is much nervous irritability and palpitation.

Directions for use: Five drops of the fluid extract in a little water three times daily.

RASPBERRY
(Rubus idaeus)

Also known as Hindleberry, Gentler berry (old names!)
Description: The raspberry can be cultivated in most temperate climates and is very common in English gardens; the canes are so well known that they need no description.
Part used:: The leaves.

Fernie says, 'The Latins named this shrub "the bramble of Ida" because it grew in abundance on that classic mountain where the shepherd Paris adjudged to Venus the prize for beauty — a golden apple on which were divinely inscribed the words. "Let it be awarded to the fairest of these womankind" '.

Dr E.D. Clarke says that the manner in which the raspberry is found in Sweden might afford useful hints as to the mode which should be adopted for its cultivation. Of all places it seems to thrive best among wood ashes and cinders, or among the ruins of houses which have been destroyed by fire. He also found it most luxuriant in those forests where the Swedes had kindled fires in the wood, and left the land strewn with the ashes of the trees. 'In the north of Sweden' he says 'neither apples, pears nor plums can be produced by cultivation but Nature has been bountiful in a profusion of wild and delicious dainties'.

'Raspberry leaves are one of the most useful and efficient remedies for women in labour, quieting untimely pains but rendering them more efficient if labour has really commenced', says an old herbalist.

Raspberry leaf tea may be taken with grateful results for several months before the expected birth. If this tea was generally used instead of the ordinary Indian variety, haemorrhage would rarely occur after confinement, and instruments would hardly ever have to be used.

It is also useful in suppressed menses especially if due to cold.

Directions for use: Add 1 pint of boiling water to 2 teaspoonsful of the leaves and infuse for five minutes. It should be taken hot as tea and may be sweetened with a little honey if desired.

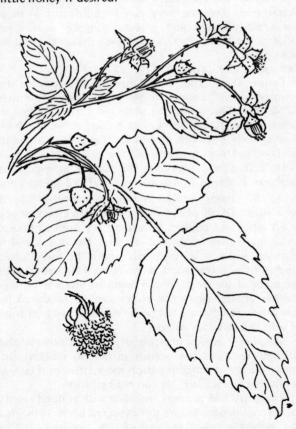

ROSEMARY
(Rosmarinus officinalis)

Also known as Romero.

Description: It is a common plant in Britain and was cultivated here prior to the Norman conquest. The stem is rather woody, square, the leaves are narrow and short, dark green above and silver below, hairy; the flowers are blue-lilac, two lipped with only two stamens. It is very aromatic.

Part used: The herb.

Gerard says, 'Rosemary groweth in France, Spaine and in other hot countries in woods and in untilled places; there is such plenty thereof in Languedocke, that the inhabitants burne scarce any other fuell; they make hedges of it in the gardens of Italy and England, being a great ornament unto the same; it groweth neither in the fields nor gardens of the Easterne cold countries but is carefully and curiously kept in pots, set into the stoves and cellers, against the injuries of their cold winters'.

Rosemary was entwined in the wreath worn by the bride at the altar in olden times, being first dipped in scented water. A wife of Henry VIII, Anne of Cleves, wore such a wreath at her wedding; and if they could afford it, a richly gilded rosemary branch was presented to each wedding guest by the parents of the bride.

Salmon says, 'Rosemary is good for diseases of the womb, coldness and weakness of the womb, whites and other distempers of those parts. It opens obstructions of the womb, provokes urine and the terms and facilitates both birth and afterbirth'.

Culpeper says, 'Both the flowers and leaves are very profitable for the whites, if they be taken daily'.

This herb is excellent for all women's ailments. It

helps to regulate menses; and should be thought of when there are pains from the uterus followed by haemorrhage. It is a good tonic for the reproductive organs.

A tea made from this herb should be taken freely by all women suffering from any menstrual troubles.

Directions for use: Put a teaspoonful of the dried herb into a teapot and fill up with boiling water (about 1½ pints). Allow to stand for five minutes and then drink as tea. It may be sweetened with honey or brown sugar if desired.

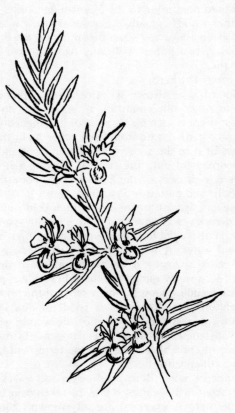

RUE
(Ruta graveolens)

Also known as Garden rue, Herb of Grace, Herbygrass, Ave-grass.

Description: This plant grows into a sturdy little shrub that is very hardy, on poor soil in many English gardens. It is bushy with small leaves of soft bluish-green, and has small yellow flowers at the top of the stems. It is one of the 'bitter' herbs and has a very aromatic scent.

Part used: The herb.

The name *Ruta* is from the Greek *reuo* to set free, because this herb is so efficacious in many diseases.

Rue constituted one of the chief ingredients of the famous antidote of Mithridates to poisons, and it was Pompey who found the formula in the satchel of the conquered king.

Fernie tells us that in olden days this plant was thought to bestow second sight; it was held so sacred at one time in these islands that missionaries sprinkled their holy water from brushes made from rue; and so it was named 'Herb of Grace'.

Gerard says, 'The garden rue, which is better than the wild rue for physic's use, grows most profitably (as Dioscorides said) under a fig tree'.

We read in *Potter's New Cyclopaedia*, 'Rue was believed to possess the merits of dispelling infection and to this day the old custom of strewing the courts with herbs (of which rue is an ingredient) is maintained'.

It is extremely useful in the suppression of menses and is a very good regulator of periods. It should be given when menses are irregular, with leucorrhoea, and the sufferer has bouts of hysteria. It helps to clear up corrosive leucorrhoea after irregular or suppressed menses.

This herb should not be taken in large doses.

Directions for use: A small wineglassful of the infusion, made by pouring 1 pint of water on to 1 oz. of the herb and allowing it to stand for a few minutes, should be taken three times daily.

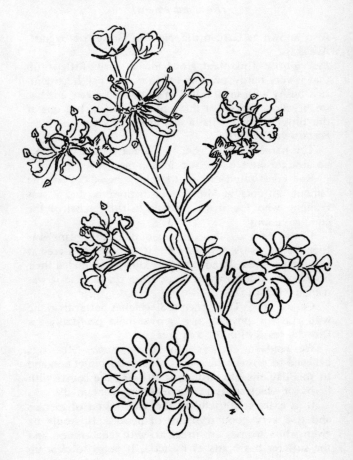

SAFFRON
(Crocus sativa)

Also known as Crocus, Alicante saffron, Valencia saffron, Hay saffron, Gatinais saffron.

Description: The plant that produces the true saffron has a round bulbous root, like a nutmeg, flat at the bottom, from which spring several white fibres; and from this root rise the flowers which have six long roundish-pointed purple petals enclosing three stamens of bright yellow.

Part used: Flower pistils.

This plant was cultivated in England in the reign of Edward the Third. It is said that a pilgrim then brought from the Levant the first root of saffron concealed in an hollow staff, at the peril of his life, and he planted it at Saffron Walden in Essex, whence the place has derived its name.

An ounce of saffron is said to require the stigmas from over 4,300 flowers so that it has always been an expensive product, and a valuable crop.

Gerard says, 'The chives steeped in water serve to illumine or (as we say) limne pictures and imagerie, as also to colour sundry meats and confections'.

Salmon says, 'It provokes urine and the Terms, facilitates the Birth and brings away the After-Birth, and causes a due cleansing'.

This is an excellent herb in the treatment of amenorrhoea (absence of menses) and dysmenorrhoea (painful and difficult menses). It will arrest chronic discharges of blood from the uterus and helps considerably when periods are excessive with dark clots. In fact it is a good regulator, increasing the menstrual flow when necessary and checking it when too excessive,

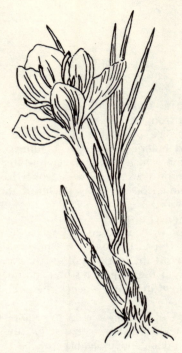

especially when any of these symptoms are due to cold. For excessive menstruation or flooding the fluid extract should be used.

Saffron also helps women who are going through the menopause when they suffer from headaches and a feeling of heat on top of the head.

Directions for use: An infusion is made by pouring 1 pint of boiling water on to 1 teaspoonful of saffron. This should be strained when cold and a teaspoonful taken three times daily.

If the fluid extract is used 4 or 5 drops should be taken in water every three or four hours until there is an improvement.

SAGE
(Salvia officinalis)

Also known as Garden sage.

Description: Growing about 2 feet tall it has hairy stems with long rough leaves, greyish green, which release an aromatic smell when handled. The flowers are a brilliant blue.

It is found on grassy downlands and where the soil is calcareous, and it now grows in many herb and country gardens.

Part used: The leaves.

One old herbalist writes, 'This excellent herb taken in any way, and for any disease, must do good, because it strengthens the head and nerves, cures trembling of the limbs and promotes a strong circulation of the fluids'.

Culpeper says, 'A decoction of the leaves and branches made and drank provokes urine, expels the dead child, brings down women's courses and causeth the hair to become black'.

Fernie says that a strong infusion of the herb has been used with success to dry up the breast milk for weaning.

Sage is a very useful remedy in the treatment of obstructed menstruation (amenorrhoea), and in menorrhalgia, flooding. In addition, it will increase menses when too scanty and check them when they are too profuse. In other words this herb is another regulator of the menses.

Directions for use: Sage tea is delicious and should be taken instead of the ordinary Indian or China varieties. Pour 1 pint of boiling water on to two teaspoonsful of the dried leaves in a teapot. Put on the lid and allow to infuse for five minutes. This tea may be sweetened with a little honey or brown sugar if desired.

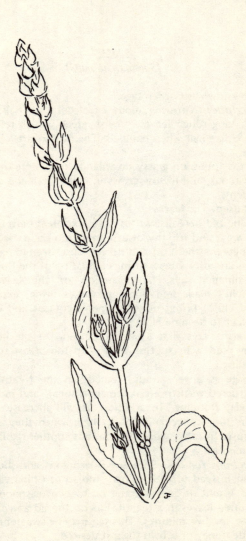

SHEPHERD'S PURSE
(Capsella bursa-pastoris)

Also known as Shepherd's Sprout, Mother's heart, Pick-pocket, Clapper's Pouch, Rattle Pouch.

Description: This is one of the most common wayside English weeds, but it grows also in most parts of the world. It has a rosette of leaves, deeply serrated on the ground level and a slender stem 10-15 inches tall bearing a spike of small, white flowers, followed by triangular flattened seed pods.

Part used: The whole plant.

Culpeper says, 'It helps all fluxes of blood caused by either inward or outward wounds; as also flux of the belly and bloody flux, spitting and voiding of blood, and stops the terms in women'.

Fernie says, 'This herb and its seed were employed in former times to promote the regular monthly flow in women'.

Bombelon, a French chemist, has praised this herb for the prompt way it arrests bleeding and floodings when given in the form of the fluid extract.

And we find in Gerard's Herbal, 'Shepheards purse staieth bleeding in any part of the body, whether the juice of the decoction thereof be drunke, or whether it be used pultesse wise, or in the bath or any other way'.

This is an excellent uterine remedy. It helps to control too frequent and copious menses, with or without quite violent colic, and it works well when every alternate period is very profuse. It is excellent when there is leucorrhoea before and after each period which is dark and offensive.

Directions for use: An infusion is made by adding 1 pint of boiling water to 1 oz. of the dried or fresh herb; this should be strained when cold and a wineglassful taken three or four times daily.

The fluid extract may be purchased and in acute cases 5 drops in water should be taken every four hours for one week and then 6 drops in water night and morning for a further two or three weeks.

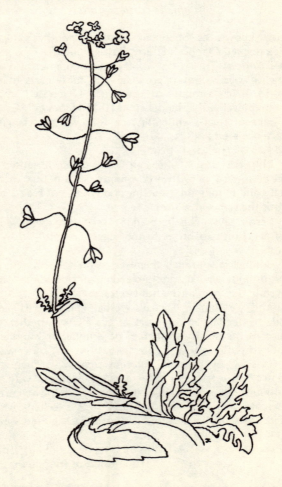

WILD THYME
(Thymus serpyllum)

Also known as Brotherwort, Creeping thyme, Mother thyme.

Description: It grows on hills, heaths and in meadows and is a creeping evergreen. This plant has a small, stringy, creeping root from which rise a great number of very slender, woody stalks having two small, roundish, green leaves, set at a joint on short footstalks. The flowers grow on the top of the stalks among the leaves, in small loose spikes of reddish purple colour. The leaves and flowers have a very sweet scent. The appearance of this herb differs slightly in different soils — some leaves may be dark green and others more hairy.

Part used: The herb.

In Greece this plant was very highly esteemed for its medicinal qualities; it was also an emblem of bravery and activity; and the ladies of long ago embroidered on the scarves which they presented to their knights, a bee hovering about a sprig of thyme, so teaching the union of the amiable and the active!

Bacon in his essay on gardens, recommends the setting out of whole walks of thyme for the pleasure of its perfume when trodden on.

Thyme is one of the most used of the culinary herbs, and today it grows in many gardens. Until very recently country folk used to drink quantities of thyme tea which has a lovely flavour.

The name mother thyme comes from its influence on the womb, an organ which the older writers always referred to as 'Mother'.

This herb is very good when the infusion is taken hot last thing at night for suppression of the menses.

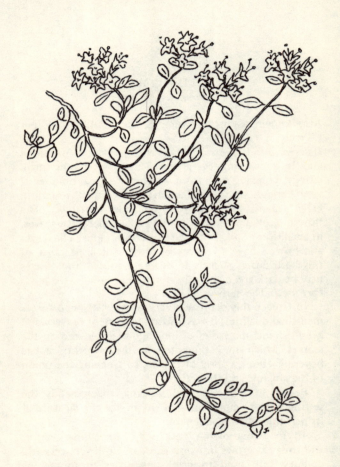

Directions for use: Pour 1 pint of boiling water on to 1 oz. of the herb and allow it to infuse for six or seven minutes. Drink hot at bedtime.

To make a tea, put a good teaspoonful of the herb into a teapot (about 1½ pints) and add boiling water. Let it stand for five minutes and then drink as tea.

YARROW
(Achillea millefolium)

Also known as Milfoil, Thousand-leaf, Nosebleed, Old man's pepper, Soldier's Woundwort, Knyghten.

Description: It is very common growing on grassy banks and meadows on a rough, downy stem 12 to 15 inches tall. The leaves are long and 1 inch broad bi-pinnate, the dark green leaflets cut into hair-like strips (feather-like). The flowers are either pink or white, very small in flat terminal clusters.

Part used: The herb.

The name Yarrow is a corruption of the Greek hiera, holy herb, because it possessed many medical properties. The name Achillea was given because the Greek warrior Achilles is said to have disclosed its virtues which had been taught to him by Chiron, the Centaur.

Fernie tells us, '. . . a charmed packet containing dried yarrow has been credited with bringing success to its bearer if at the same time he were admitted to the knowledge of a traditional secret (only whispered to the initiated), and that this was the first herb our Saviour had put into His hand when a child'.

Professor Burnett remarks, 'It is little esteemed except by the good women of the Orkneys who hold Milfoil tea in high repute for its power in dispelling melancholy'.

Yarrow has stimulating and astringent qualities, it is very positive but slow in action. Its chief influence is felt in the renal and pelvic organs and it is a most useful medicine in the treatment of leucorrhoea. Through its astringent property it helps to stem profuse menstruation when a warm infusion or tea should be taken.

Directions for use: A pint of boiling water should be

poured on to 1 oz. of the dried herb and strained when cold, and a wineglassful taken three times daily.

A tea is made by pouring a pint of boiling water on to 2 teaspoonsful of the herb and after five minutes this should be taken as tea.

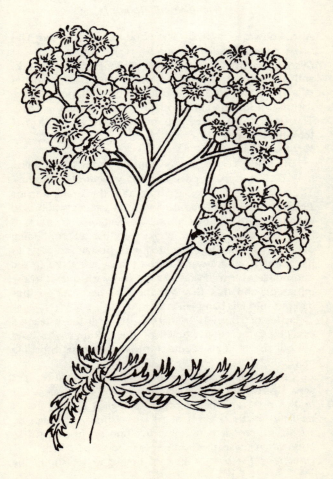

SUPPLEMENTARY ADVICE

All too often the diet of patients complaining of menstrual troubles, needs adjusting.

No practitioner is popular if interference with daily food is mentioned and yet good, wholesome, natural and balanced meals are more important today than ever before, because so much of our foodstuffs contain little or no nutriment, and should be avoided.

Many troubles are caused by the intake of too many carbohydrates and starches. Cakes, pastry, biscuits and puddings should be reduced to the minimum.

Bread should be made from compost grown 100 per cent. wholemeal flour and if this cannot be tolerated for reasons of ulceration, etc., then 81 or 85 per cent. extraction is the next best thing.

Most people take far too much sugar, particularly the white varieties. White sugar sweetens food but has no nutritive value; it is very acid and puts a strain on the digestive and eliminative organs. A little honey may be taken with advantage and if sugar must be used, then barbados is the best but it should be taken as sparingly as possible.

A salad should be taken every day, consisting of as many of the following ingredients that are available: lettuce, shredded white cabbage, grated raw carrot and beetroot, cucumber, tomatoes, watercress, mustard and cress, celery, endive, raw mushrooms, peppers and spring onions. Delicious dishes can be made by adding some French dressing and either cottage or cream cheese with added chives, grated cheddar cheese or chopped nuts as protein. To complete this meal fresh fruit should follow.

One hot meal daily should consist of a little lamb,

chicken or fish with two or three conservatively cooked vegetables including at least one green vegetable. If potatoes are taken they should be cooked in their jackets, as mineral salts are to be found just beneath the thin top skin, and if the potatoes are peeled these are lost. If you are a vegetarian then an omelette or one of the vegetarian savoury dishes with vegetables given in many books, makes a balanced meal.

Herbal teas described earlier in the book should replace Indian tea and coffee. The intake of milk should be cut to the minimum, particularly by those who suffer from leucorrhoea, as this is mucus-forming.

The following items should be avoided: spicy foods, salted fish, pickles, all fried foods, salt bacon, curry, pork, vinegar and pepper.

Two vitamins helpful to women are the B complex and E. Natural, rather than synthetic vitamins are obtainable from health food stores.

The most important foods containing the B vitamins are: dried brewers' yeast, wheatgerm, soya beans, calves' liver, dried skimmed milk, brazil nuts, sunflower seed oil, cashew nuts, egg yolk, walnuts, oatmeal, whole wheat meal, molasses, almonds, brown rice and turnip tops.

Vitamin E should be taken regularly by young women who cannot conceive as it is known as the 'fertility vitamin' and will very often solve this problem. It is also very helpful at the time of the menopause.

Foods richest in Vitamin E are wheatgerm oil, soya bean oil, maize oil, eggs, lamb, butter, brown rice, turnip tops and green peas.

Foods rich in iron are especially good for women as anaemia can cause all kinds of menstrual troubles and some of the following should be included in at least one meal every day: kidneys, liver, eggs, bran, dried peaches, molasses, peas, oatmeal, raisins, green vegetables, dried fruits, whole cereals, jacket potatoes, cabbage, white fish and apples.

Calcium is important because if the level drops at the

beginning of menstruation, as it does if extra doses are not taken into the body, the muscular walls of the uterus go into spasms of cramp thus causing pain. And again at the time of the menopause, when the body is readjusting, there is a lack of ovarian hormones which cause severe calcium deficiency. Calcium tablets will help to ease the tensions, hot flushes and all the other prevalent symptoms at these times.

Foods rich in Calcium are nearly all the cheeses (except the highly flavoured varieties), dried whole and skimmed milk, whitebait, sardines, turnip tops, figs, dried apricots, soya beans, kale, watercress, sole, eggs, wheat bran, cauliflower, molasses, apples, walnuts, brown rice, peanut butter, dates, celery, salmon and raisins.

All aluminium cooking utensils should be replaced by those made of stainless steel, enamel and pyrex oven-ware.

Herbs should never be boiled or infused in aluminium pans as this metal is detrimental to health.

Most women do not take sufficient exercise in the fresh air. Chores in the home do not replace a brisk walk which should be taken every day, if health is to be maintained. Obviously strenuous exercise and over-stretching are not desirable but most people would do well to think how little walking is done today when so many cars take people everywhere they wish to go!

A few simple rhythmical exercises in front of an open window, with some deep breathing would be beneficial.

Posture is all important and women should 'walk tall' easily and rhythmically. Standing for too long is not good, and stretching up to peg clothes on to a line that is too high should be avoided.

Remember that hot baths can be enervating and these should be taken warm, not hot, followed by a brisk rub with a rough towel.

By taking the appropriate herbal remedies and following the advice in this section, some improvement should be noticed in a short time.

THERAPEUTIC INDEX

Afterbirth, to expel, Angelica.
Childbirth, for easier, Raspberry.
Headache with menses, Feverfew.
Headache from suppressed menses, Peppermint.
Hysteria, Arrach, Feverfew, Rue.
Leucorrhoea, Black cohosh, Pulsatilla, Rue, Yarrow.
Menopause, Lady's slipper, Pulsatilla, Saffron.
Menses, absent, Saffron.
Menses, cessation of, Peppermint.
Menses, delayed, Balm.
Menses, flooding, Saffron, Sage.
Menses, too frequent, Shepherd's purse.
Menses, irregular, Black cohosh, Mugwort, Rosemary, Rue.
Menses, irregular with leucorrhoea, Rue.
Menses, obstructed, Mugwort, Sage.
Menses, too profuse, Angelica, Arrach, Black horehound, Saffron, Sage, Shepherd's purse, Yarrow.
Menses, scanty, Black cohosh, Fennel, Motherwort, Pulsatilla
Menses, suppressed, Angelica, Arrach, Balm, Basil, Black Cohosh, Black horehound, Feverfew, Motherwort, Mugwort, Raspberry, Rue, Sage, Wild thyme.
Menstruation, difficult, Catmint, Cramp bark, Pulsatilla, Saffron.
Nervous agitation prior to menses, Catmint.
Nervous irritability, Motherwort, Pulsatilla.
Neuralgia in pelvic region, Black cohosh.
Pains, bearing down, Cramp bark, Motherwort.
Pains, cramping before menses, Lady's slipper.
Pains, cramping during menses, Cramp bark, Lady's slipper, Motherwort, Pulsatilla.

Pains, cramping of pregnancy, Cramp bark.

Pains of labour, Black horehound, Motherwort, Raspberry.

Pains from menses suppressed, Peppermint.

Pains before menses, Balm.

Pains from delayed menses, Basil.

Pains during menses, Balm, Mugwort.

Pains in uterus, followed by haemorrhage, Rosemary.

Pains in uterus, neuralgic, Cramp bark.

Pains in uterus, rheumatic, Black cohosh.

Prolapse of uterus, Black cohosh, Motherwort, Pulsatilla.

Tonic for generative organs, Motherwort, Rosemary.

Tonic for uterine membranes, Motherwort.